PREDIABETES DIET PLAN FOR WEIGHT LOSS

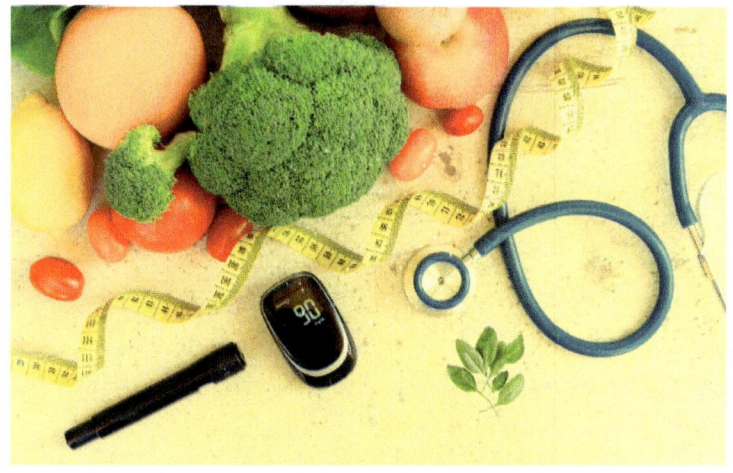

Reverse and Prevent Diabetes through Healthy Meal Recipes

Martins Food

DISCLAIMER

The author holds the copyright to this work. No part of this publication may be reproduced, distributed, or transmitted in any form or by any means, including photocopying, recording, or other electronic or mechanical methods, without the prior written permission of the author, except in the case of brief quotations embodied in critical reviews and certain other noncommercial uses permitted by copyright law.

All rights reserved. The unauthorized reproduction or distribution of this copyrighted work is illegal and may result in civil or criminal penalties in accordance with applicable copyright laws. The publisher and author assume no responsibility for the use or misuse of the information contained within this book.

TABLE OF CONTENTS

INTRODUCTION
CHAPTER 1: OVERVIEW OF PREDIABETES
BREAKFAST RECIPES:
Berry-Kefir Smoothie
Apple-Cinnamon Overnight Oats
Sriracha, Egg & Avocado Overnight Oats
Berry-Orange Chia Pudding
Spinach-Avocado Smoothie
Blueberry Almond Chia Pudding
Cocoa-Chia Pudding with Raspberries
Breakfast Carrot-Cake Oatmeal Cakes
Strawberry & Cream Cheese Oatmeal Cakes
Zucchini Banana Bread
CHAPTER 2: LUNCH RECIPES
Winter Kale & Quinoa Salad with Avocado
Classic Sesame Noodles with Chicken
Fresh Sweet Corn Salad
Sheet-Pan Chicken Fajita Bowls
Vegetable Weight-Loss Soup
Beef & Bean Sloppy Joes
Chipotle-Lime Cauliflower Taco Bowls
Vegetarian Stuffed Cabbage
Chicken Chili Verde
Chickpea & Potato Curry

CHAPTER 3: DINNER RECIPES

Gochujang-Glazed Salmon with Garlic Spinach

Chopped Salad with Chicken & Creamy Chipotle Dressing

Lemongrass Pork & Spaghetti Squash Noodle Bowl with Peanut Sauce

Kale & Avocado Salad with Blueberries & Edamame

Teriyaki Chicken Skillet Casserole with Broccoli

Spicy Shrimp Tacos

Roasted Brussels Sprout & Butternut Squash Salad

Slow-Cooker Chicken Chili

Chicken Enchilada Skillet Casserole

Sheet-Pan Balsamic-Parmesan Roasted Chickpeas & Vegetables

28 DAYS MEAL PLAN

CONVERSION TABLE

INTRODUCTION

Welcome to the Prediabetes Diet Plan for Weight Loss, where a delightful array of dishes awaits you! Explore a wonderful selection of meals packed with fiber and protein, while keeping carbs moderate and saturated fat low.

Start your day with nourishing breakfast options like Berry-Kefir Smoothie . Our collection of 10 wholesome Breakfast features Apple-Cinnamon Overnight Oats, Cocoa-Chia pudding with Raspberries, and Zucchini Banana Bread.

Craving a refreshing salad? Choose from our mouthwatering options such as kale and Avocado Salad with BlueBerries and Red Onions, winter Kale and Quinoa Salad with Avocado, and Fresh Sweet Corn Salad. For satisfying lunches, indulge in vegetable Weight-Loss Soup, Vegetarian Stuffed Cabbage or Chicken Chili Verde.

Dinner becomes a culinary adventure with dishes like Spicy Shrimp Tacos, Slow-Cooker Chicken Chili, and Lemongrass Pork and Spaghetti Squash Noodle Bowl with Peanut Sauce. all tailored to meet your dietary needs.

We've carefully curated recipes with ingredients associated with positive benefits for those with prediabetes, ensuring you have the healthiest year yet! Get ready to savor every moment in the kitchen, as you embark on this journey to wellness. Happy cooking!

Martins Food

WELCOME

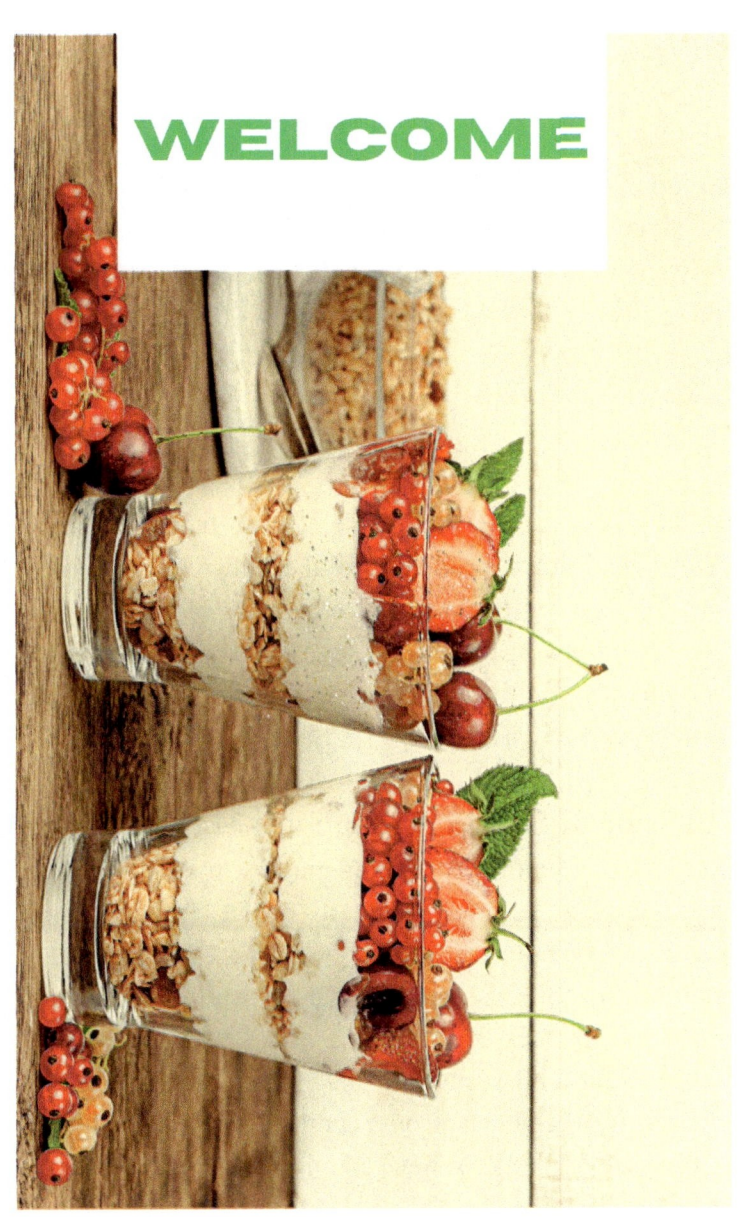

CHAPTER 1: OVERVIEW OF PREDIABETES

Are you aware that your blood sugar levels are elevated but haven't reached the diabetic threshold? You might be experiencing prediabetes. Prediabetes is characterized by higher-than-normal blood sugar levels, though not yet at the level of type 2 diabetes. The encouraging news is that you can reverse this condition through lifestyle adjustments.

The key to reversing prediabetes lies in tackling insulin resistance. Insulin, produced by the pancreas, facilitates the transfer of blood sugar from the bloodstream into cells for energy usage. When sugar fails to enter cells, it accumulates in the bloodstream, potentially causing harm to the body over time.

The Role of Diet in Prediabetes Management:
Diet plays a pivotal role in managing prediabetes. An unhealthy diet can contribute to obesity, a significant risk factor for both prediabetes and type 2 diabetes. This is because obesity exacerbates insulin resistance. Research indicates that shedding about 5 to 7 percent of body weight, and sustaining that weight loss, can slash the risk of prediabetes progression to type 2 diabetes by a remarkable 58%. When coupled with at least 150

minutes of weekly exercise, the likelihood of developing type 2 diabetes decreases even further.

What are the optimal food choices for individuals with prediabetes?

Prediabetes entails a degree of insulin resistance, complicating the body's carbohydrate processing. A straightforward approach to supporting your body involves substituting high-carb options like white rice, potatoes, and white bread with fiber-rich unrefined alternatives such as brown rice, whole grain breads, whole grain cereals, and vegetables. These nutrient-dense foods have a lower impact on blood sugar levels and can facilitate weight loss while maintaining stable blood sugar levels.

Studies have demonstrated that individuals who consume a moderate amount of carbohydrates (approximately 150g per day) and opt for foods with a lower glycemic impact experience reduced postprandial glucose levels, irrespective of weight loss, compared to those on high-carb diets.

When managing weight, the method of food preparation also warrants attention. Limiting the use of butter or oil for frying onions, sautéing vegetables, mashing potatoes, or scrambling eggs can lower the overall calorie intake of a meal. Moreover, it's crucial to restrict fats and oils added to foods before consumption, such as butter, margarine, cream cheese, and salad dressings, as they often contain high levels of fat, added sugar, and salt, while being low in dietary fiber.

What are the optimal food choices for individuals with prediabetes?

For those with prediabetes, shedding excess weight and adhering to a moderate carbohydrate diet are crucial steps to stave off the onset of type 2 diabetes. Equally important is reducing the consumption of saturated fats, as these fats are calorie-dense and can adversely affect blood lipid levels, increasing the risk of heart disease, a prevalent cause of mortality in the UK. To decrease saturated fat intake, consider substituting vegetarian sources of protein for meat, particularly red meat. Excellent protein alternatives include soy, tempeh, tofu, beans, and lentils.

A recommended dietary guideline suggests that the total fat content of a meal should not exceed 18%, with only 5% comprising saturated fat. Hence, in a 100g serving, saturated fat should not exceed 5g out of a total fat content of 18g. Prediabetic individuals are advised to limit their daily carbohydrate intake to 150g, which should constitute approximately 45% of their daily calorie consumption.

Some studies propose that transitioning to a vegetarian diet following a prediabetes diagnosis may be beneficial. While not obligatory, reducing meat consumption a few times a week and opting for fish or vegetarian alternatives can help lower weekly calorie intake and alleviate the body's inflammation and insulin resistance.

BREAKFAST RECIPES:

Berry-Kefir Smoothie

Enhance your morning with a probiotic kick by incorporating kefir into your smoothie. Feel at liberty to utilize any berries and nut butter available for this nutritious smoothie recipe.

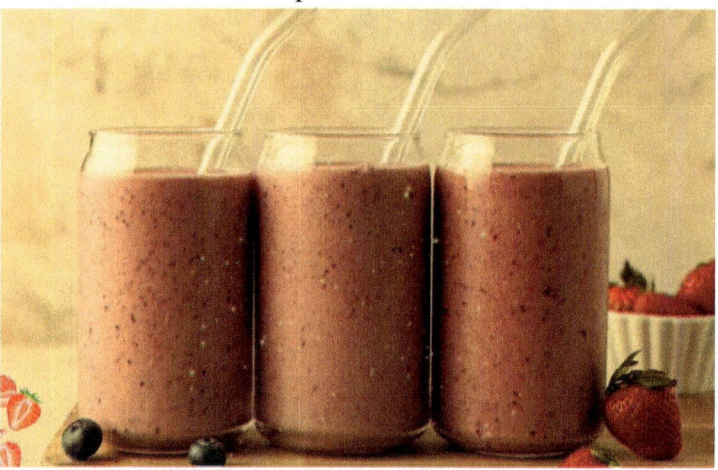

Preparation Time:5 minutes
Total Time:5 minutes
Servings:1
Yield:1 serving

Nutrition Profile:
High in Calcium, Suitable for Healthy Pregnancy, Soy-Free, Vegetarian, High-Protein, Egg-Free, Gluten-Free, Low-Calorie

Ingredients:
- 1 ½ cups frozen mixed berries
- 1 cup plain kefir
- ½ medium banana
- 2 teaspoons almond butter
- ½ teaspoon vanilla extract

Directions:
1. In a blender, combine frozen berries, kefir, banana, almond butter, and vanilla extract.
2. Blend the ingredients until smooth.

Apple-Cinnamon Overnight Oats

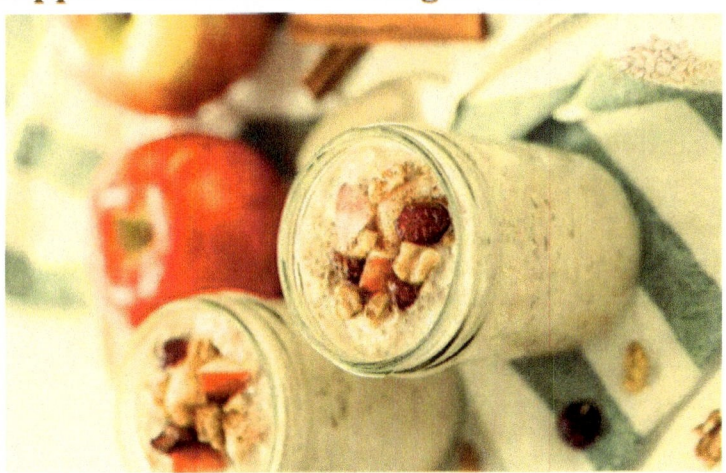

Preparation Time:10 minutes
Additional Time:5 hours 50 minutes
Total Time:6 hours

Servings:1
Yield:1 serving

Nutrition Profile:
Dairy-Free, Soy-Free, Vegan, Vegetarian, Egg-Free, Gluten-Free, Low-Calorie

Ingredients:
- ½ cup old-fashioned rolled oats
- ½ cup unsweetened almond milk
- ½ tablespoon chia seeds (optional)
- 1 teaspoon maple syrup
- ¼ teaspoon ground cinnamon
- Pinch of salt
- ½ cup diced apple
- 2 tablespoons toasted pecans (optional)

Directions:
1. In a pint-sized jar, combine oats, almond milk, chia seeds (if using), maple syrup, cinnamon, and salt. Stir well to combine. Cover the jar and refrigerate overnight.
2. Before serving, top the oat mixture with diced apple and toasted pecans, if desired.

Sriracha, Egg & Avocado Overnight Oats

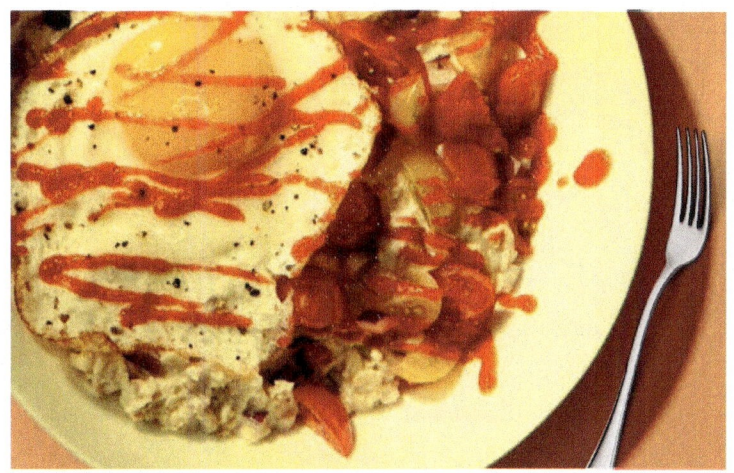

Preparation Time:15 minutes
Additional Time:7 hours 45 minutes
Total Time:8 hours
Servings:1
Yield:1 bowl

Nutrition Profile:
Dairy-Free, Promotes Healthy Aging, Low-Sodium, Low Added Sugar, Soy-Free, High-Fiber, Egg-Free, Gluten-Free, Low-Calorie

Ingredients:
- ½ cup rolled oats
- ¾ cup water
- 1 tablespoon onion
- ¼ avocado, sliced
- 2 cherry tomatoes, chopped

- 1 large egg, fried
- 1 teaspoon Sriracha

Directions:
1. In a small bowl or jar, combine rolled oats and water. Cover and refrigerate overnight.
2. Stir in the onion and microwave in 30-second intervals, stirring occasionally, until heated through.
3. Arrange the heated oats in a bowl with sliced avocado and chopped tomatoes.
4. Top with the fried egg and Sriracha.

Berry-Orange Chia Pudding

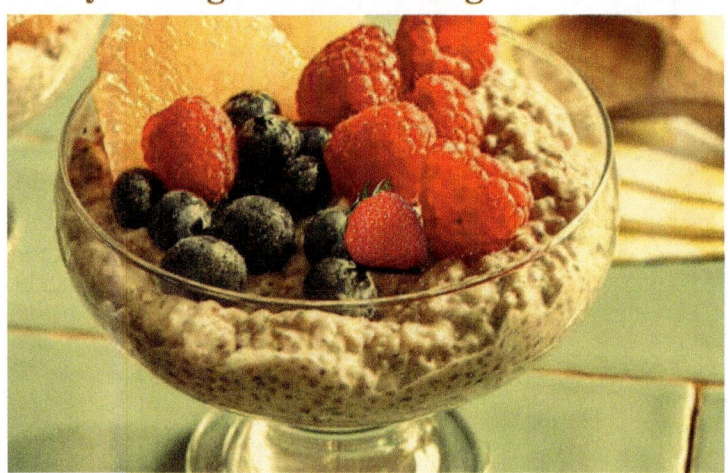

Active Time:10 minutes
Total Time:8 hours 10 minutes

Servings:4

Nutrition Profile:
Suitable for Diabetes, Nut-Free, Dairy-Free, Soy-Free, High-Fiber, Vegan, Vegetarian, Egg-Free, Gluten-Free, Low-Calorie

Ingredients:
- 1 (14 ounce) can of coconut milk
- 1 cup mixed berries
- ½ cup orange juice
- ½ cup chia seeds
- 2 tablespoons pure maple syrup

Directions:
1. In a blender, combine coconut milk, mixed berries, and orange juice. Blend until smooth.
2. Transfer the mixture to a container and stir in chia seeds and maple syrup.
3. Cover the container and refrigerate overnight.

Spinach-Avocado Smoothie

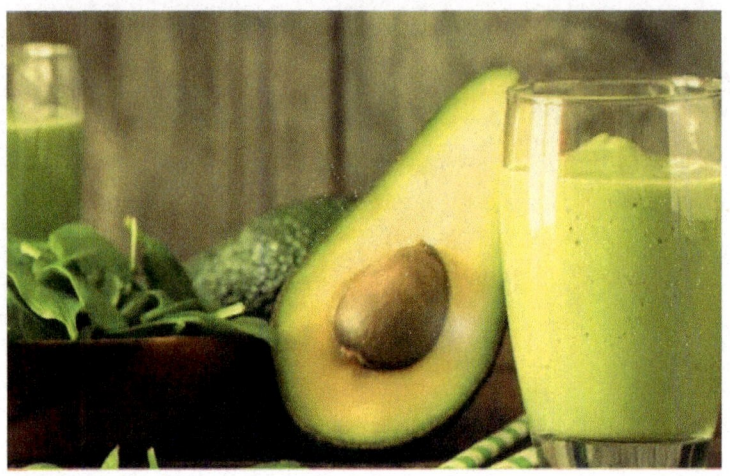

Preparation Time:5 minutes
Total Time:5 minutes
Servings:1
Yield:2 cups

Nutrition Profile:
Rich in Calcium for Bone Health, Nut-Free, Suitable for Healthy Pregnancy, Promotes Healthy Aging, Supports Healthy Immunity, Low in Sodium, Suitable for High Blood Pressure, Soy-Free, High in Fiber, Heart-Healthy, Vegetarian, Egg-Free, Gluten-Free, Low in Calories

Ingredients:
- 1 cup nonfat plain yogurt
- 1 cup fresh spinach
- 1 frozen banana
- ¼ avocado

- 2 tablespoons water
- 1 teaspoon honey

Directions:
1. In a blender, combine nonfat plain yogurt, fresh spinach, frozen banana, avocado, water, and honey.
2. Blend until smooth and pureed.

Blueberry Almond Chia Pudding

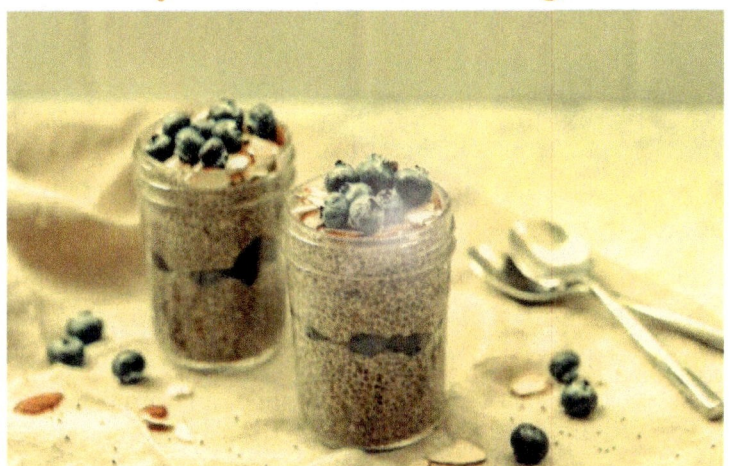

Preparation Time:10 minutes
Additional Time:8 hours
Total Time:8 hours 10 minutes
Servings:1
Yield:1 cup

Nutrition Profile:

Rich in Calcium for Bone Health, Suitable for Diabetes, Dairy-Free, Suitable for Healthy Pregnancy, Promotes Healthy Aging, Low in Sodium, Soy-Free, High in Fiber, Heart-Healthy, Vegan, Vegetarian, Egg-Free, Gluten-Free, Low in Calories

Ingredients:
- ½ cup unsweetened almond milk or other non dairy milk alternative
- 2 tablespoons chia seeds
- 2 teaspoons pure maple syrup
- ⅛ teaspoon almond extract
- ½ cup fresh blueberries, divided
- 1 tablespoon toasted slivered almonds, divided

Directions:
1. In a small bowl, mix together the unsweetened almond milk (or other non dairy milk alternative), chia seeds, maple syrup, and almond extract. Cover the bowl and refrigerate for a minimum of 8 hours or up to 3 days.
2. When ready to serve, stir the pudding thoroughly. Spoon approximately half of the pudding into a serving glass or bowl and layer with half of the blueberries and almonds. Add the remaining pudding and top with the rest of the blueberries and almonds.

Cocoa-Chia Pudding with Raspberries

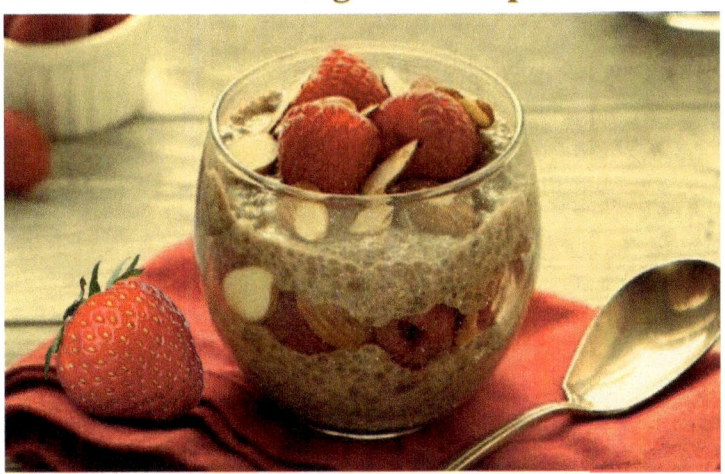

Preparation Time:10 minutes
Additional Time:8 hours
Total Time:8 hours 10 minutes
Servings:1
Yield:1 cup

Nutrition Profile:
Rich in Calcium for Bone Health, Suitable for Diabetes, Dairy-Free, Suitable for Healthy Pregnancy, Promotes Healthy Aging, Supports Healthy Immunity, Low in Sodium, Soy-Free, High in Fiber, Heart-Healthy, Vegan, Vegetarian, Egg-Free, Gluten-Free, Low in Calories

Ingredients:
- ½ cup unsweetened almond milk or another non dairy milk alternative

- 2 tablespoons chia seeds
- 2 teaspoons pure maple syrup
- ½ teaspoon unsweetened cocoa powder
- ¼ teaspoon vanilla extract
- ½ cup fresh raspberries, divided
- 1 tablespoon toasted sliced almonds, divided

Directions:
1. In a small bowl, combine the unsweetened almond milk (or another non dairy milk alternative), chia seeds, maple syrup, cocoa powder, and vanilla extract. Cover the bowl and refrigerate for a minimum of 8 hours or up to 3 days.
2. When ready to serve, stir the mixture well. Spoon approximately half of the pudding into a serving glass or bowl and layer with half of the raspberries and almonds. Add the remaining pudding and top with the rest of the raspberries and almonds.

Breakfast Carrot-Cake Oatmeal Cakes

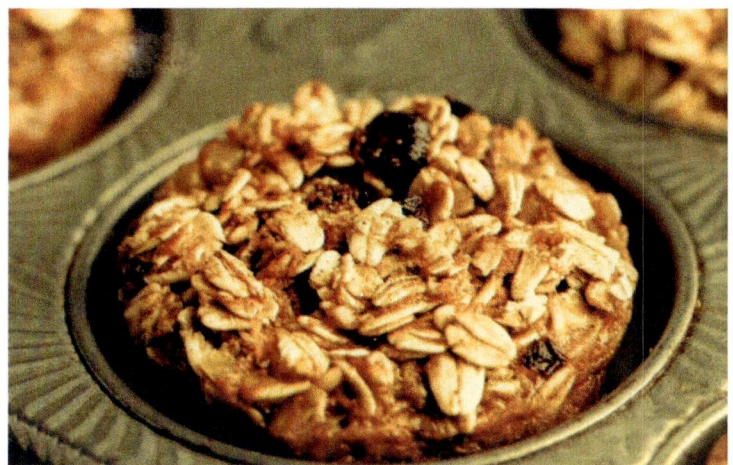

Active Time:15 minutes
Total Time:50 minutes
Servings:12

Nutrition Profile:
Suitable for Diabetes, Soy-Free, Heart-Healthy, Vegetarian, Gluten-Free

Ingredients:
- 3 cups old-fashioned rolled oats
- 1 ¼ cups low-fat milk
- ⅓ cup packed brown sugar
- ¼ cup unsweetened applesauce
- 2 large eggs, lightly beaten
- 1 tablespoon ground cinnamon
- 1 teaspoon baking powder

- 1 teaspoon vanilla extract
- ½ teaspoon ground nutmeg
- ½ teaspoon salt
- ½ cup finely shredded carrot
- ¼ cup raisins, chopped
- ¼ cup finely chopped walnuts

Directions:
1. Preheat the oven to 375°F and coat a 12-cup muffin tin with cooking spray.
2. In a large bowl, combine oats, milk, brown sugar, applesauce, eggs, cinnamon, baking powder, vanilla, nutmeg, and salt. Fold in the shredded carrot, chopped raisins, and chopped walnuts.
3. Divide the batter evenly among the prepared muffin cups, filling each about 1/3 full.
4. Bake for 25 to 30 minutes, or until a toothpick inserted in the center comes out clean.
5. Allow the oatmeal cakes to cool in the muffin tin for 10 minutes, then transfer them to a wire rack to cool further.
6. Serve the oatmeal cakes warm or at room temperature.

Strawberry & Cream Cheese Oatmeal Cakes

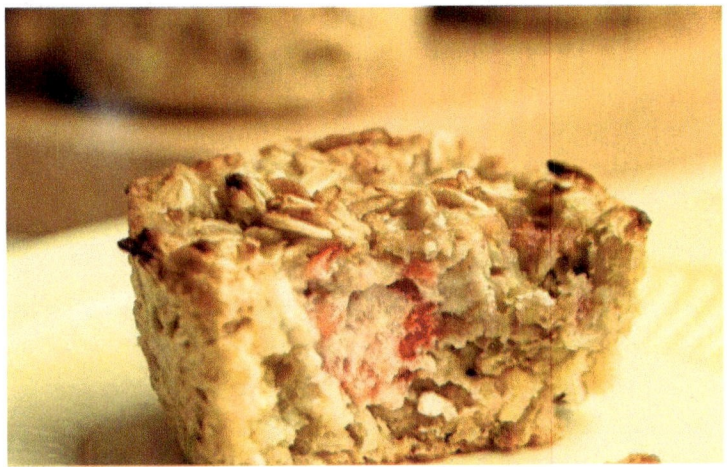

Active Time:15 minutes
Total Time:50 minutes
Servings:12

Nutrition Profile:
Suitable for Diabetes, Nut-Free, Soy-Free, Heart-Healthy, Vegetarian, Gluten-Free

Ingredients:
- ¼ cup reduced-fat cream cheese, at room temperature
- 1 tablespoon strawberry jam
- 3 cups old-fashioned rolled oats
- 1 ¼ cups low-fat milk
- ⅓ cup packed brown sugar

- ¼ cup unsweetened applesauce
- 2 large eggs, lightly beaten
- 1 teaspoon baking powder
- 1 teaspoon vanilla extract
- ½ teaspoon salt
- ¾ cup chopped fresh or frozen strawberries, divided

Directions:
1. Preheat the oven to 375°F and coat a 12-cup muffin tin with cooking spray.
2. In a small bowl, whisk together the cream cheese and strawberry jam.
3. In a large bowl, combine oats, milk, brown sugar, applesauce, eggs, baking powder, vanilla, and salt. Fold in 1/2 cup of the chopped strawberries.
4. Fill each prepared muffin cup with 2 to 3 tablespoons of batter. Top each with a dollop of the cream cheese mixture and some of the remaining 1/4 cup of chopped strawberries. Cover with the remaining batter and press slightly to compact.
5. Bake for 25 to 30 minutes, or until a toothpick inserted into the center comes out clean.
6. Allow the oatmeal cakes to cool in the muffin tin for 10 minutes. Then, run a knife around the edges of the muffin cups to release the oatmeal

cakes and transfer them to a wire rack to cool further.
7. Serve the oatmeal cakes warm or at room temperature.

Zucchini Banana Bread

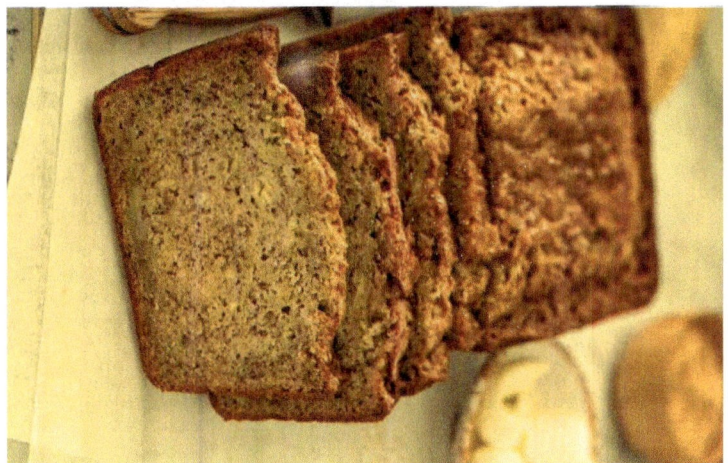

Active Time:15 minutes
Total Time:50 minutes
Servings:12

Nutrition Profile:
Suitable for Diabetes, Nut-Free, Soy-Free, Heart-Healthy, Vegetarian, Gluten-Free

Ingredients:
- ¼ cup reduced-fat cream cheese, at room temperature

- 1 tablespoon strawberry jam
- 3 cups old-fashioned rolled oats
- 1 ¼ cups low-fat milk
- ⅓ cup packed brown sugar
- ¼ cup unsweetened applesauce
- 2 large eggs, lightly beaten
- 1 teaspoon baking powder
- 1 teaspoon vanilla extract
- ½ teaspoon salt
- ¾ cup chopped fresh or frozen strawberries, divided

Directions:
1. Preheat the oven to 375°F and coat a 12-cup muffin tin with cooking spray.
2. In a small bowl, whisk together the cream cheese and strawberry jam.
3. In a large bowl, combine oats, milk, brown sugar, applesauce, eggs, baking powder, vanilla, and salt. Fold in 1/2 cup of the chopped strawberries.
4. Fill each prepared muffin cup with 2 to 3 tablespoons of batter. Top each with a dollop of the cream cheese mixture and some of the remaining 1/4 cup of chopped strawberries. Cover with the remaining batter and press slightly to compact.
5. Bake for 25 to 30 minutes, or until a toothpick inserted into the center comes out clean.

6. Allow the oatmeal cakes to cool in the muffin tin for 10 minutes. Then, run a knife around the edges of the muffin cups to release the oatmeal cakes and transfer them to a wire rack to cool further.
7. Serve the oatmeal cakes warm or at room temperature.

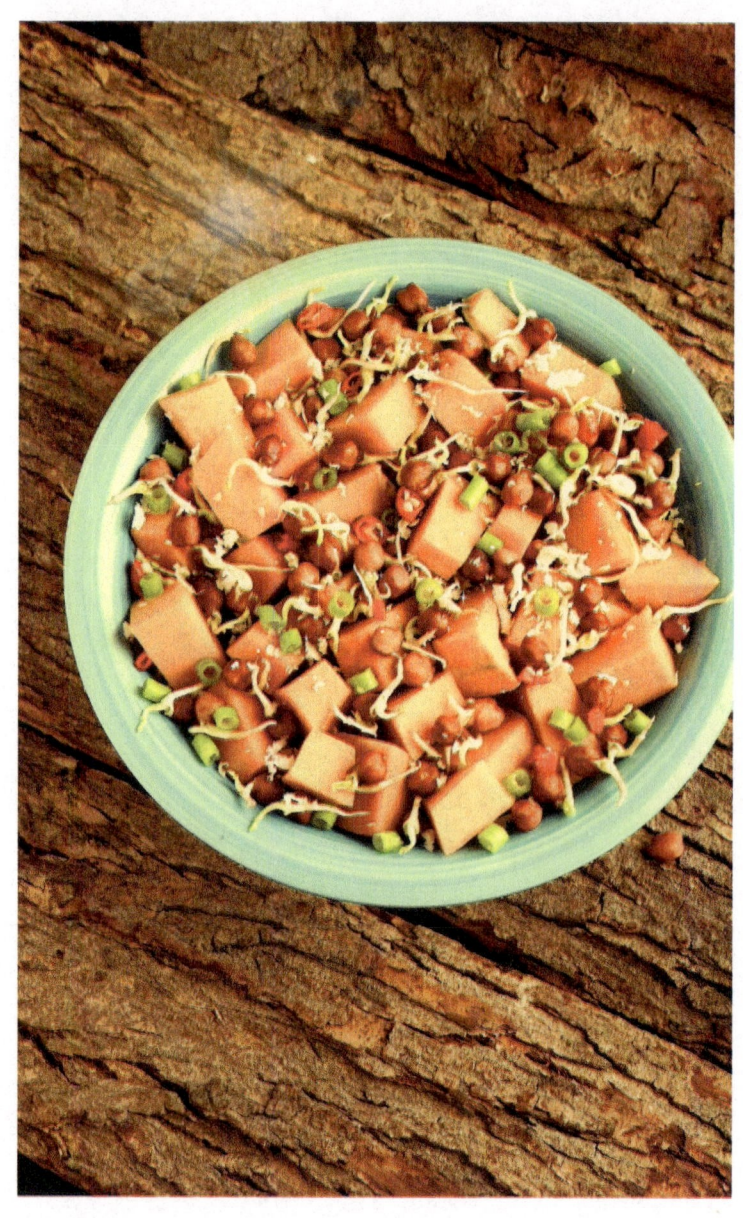

CHAPTER 2: LUNCH RECIPES

Winter Kale & Quinoa Salad with Avocado

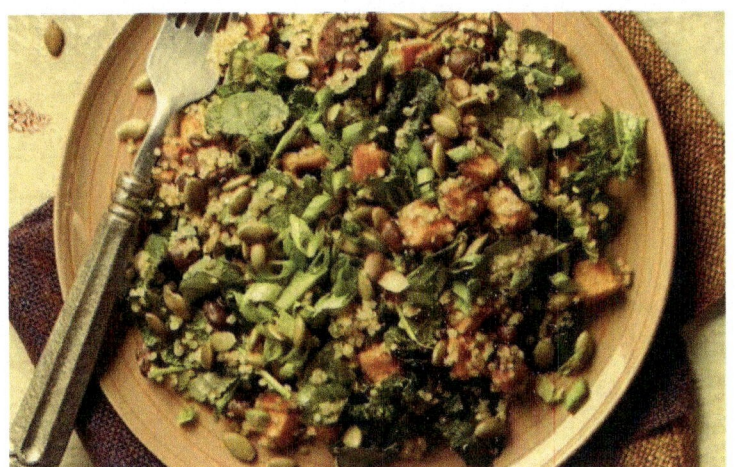

Preparation Time:15 minutes
Additional Time:20 minutes
Total Time:35 minutes
Servings:2
Yield:2 servings

Nutrition Profile:

Suitable for Diabetes, Promotes Healthy Aging, Supports Healthy Immunity, Low in Sodium, Suitable for High Blood Pressure, High in Fiber, Heart-Healthy, Low in Calories

Ingredients:
- 1 small sweet potato, peeled and diced into 1/2-inch pieces (about 1 1/2 cups)
- 2 ½ teaspoons olive oil, divided
- ½ avocado
- 1 tablespoon lime juice
- 1 clove garlic, peeled
- ½ teaspoon ground cumin
- ⅛ teaspoon salt
- ⅛ teaspoon ground pepper
- 1-2 tablespoons water
- 1 cup cooked quinoa
- ¾ cup no-salt-added canned black beans, rinsed
- 1 ½ cups chopped baby kale
- 2 tablespoons pepitas (pumpkin seeds)
- 1 scallion, chopped

Directions:
1. Preheat the oven to 400 degrees F.
2. On a large rimmed baking sheet, toss the diced sweet potato with 1 teaspoon of olive oil. Roast, stirring once halfway through, until tender, about 25 minutes.
3. Meanwhile, in a blender or food processor, combine the remaining 1 1/2 teaspoons of olive oil, avocado, lime juice, garlic, ground cumin, salt, pepper, and 1 tablespoon of water. Process

until smooth. Add 1 more tablespoon of water if needed to reach the desired consistency.
4. In a medium bowl, combine the roasted sweet potato, cooked quinoa, rinsed black beans, and chopped baby kale. Drizzle the avocado dressing over the mixture and gently toss to coat.
5. Top the salad with pepitas and chopped scallion.

Classic Sesame Noodles with Chicken

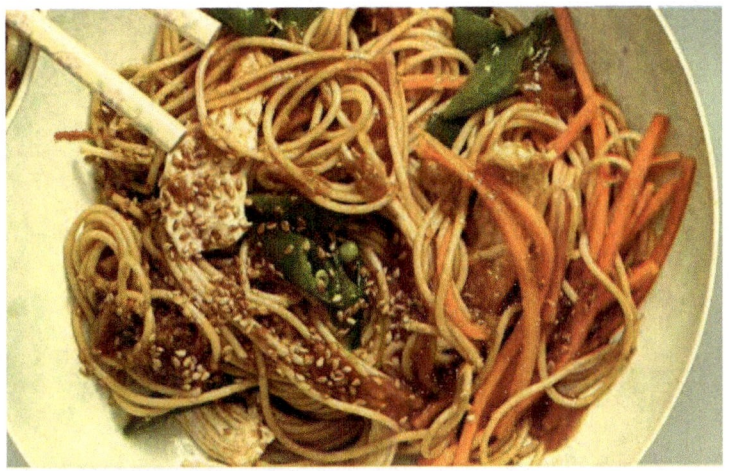

Cooking Time:20 minutes
Total Time:20 minutes
Servings:4
Yield:4 servings

Nutrition Profile:

Suitable for Diabetes, Nut-Free, Dairy-Free, Suitable for Healthy Pregnancy, Promotes Healthy Aging, Supports Healthy Immunity, Low in Sodium, Low in Added Sugar, High in Fiber, Heart-Healthy, High in Protein, Egg-Free, Low in Calories

Ingredients:
- 8 ounces whole-wheat spaghetti
- 3 tablespoons toasted (dark) sesame oil
- 2 scallions, chopped
- 1 tablespoon minced garlic
- 2 teaspoons minced fresh ginger
- 1 teaspoon brown sugar
- 2 tablespoons reduced-sodium soy sauce
- 2 tablespoons ketchup
- 8 ounces cooked boneless, skinless chicken breast, shredded
- 1 cup julienned carrots
- 1 cup sliced snap peas
- 3 tablespoons toasted sesame seeds

Directions:

1. Cook the spaghetti in a pot of boiling water according to the package instructions. Drain, rinse, and transfer to a large bowl.
2. In a small saucepan, combine the toasted sesame oil, chopped scallions, minced garlic, minced

fresh ginger, and brown sugar. Heat over medium heat until it starts to sizzle. Cook for about 15 seconds. Remove from heat and stir in the reduced-sodium soy sauce and ketchup. Add this mixture to the noodles along with the shredded chicken, julienned carrots, sliced snap peas, and toasted sesame seeds. Gently toss to combine.

Fresh Sweet Corn Salad

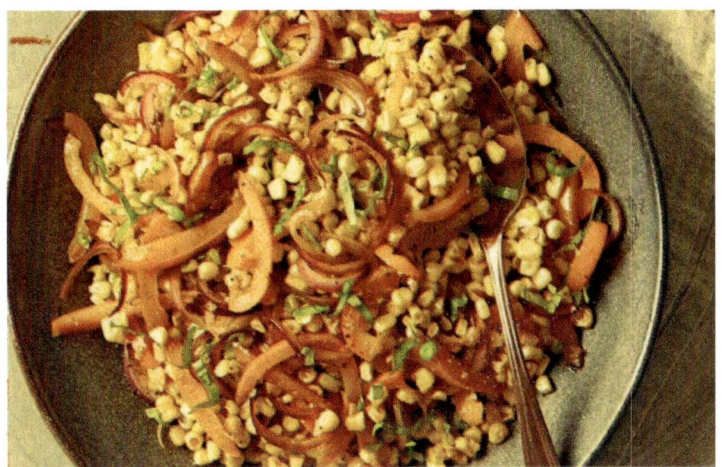

Preparation Time:10 minutes
Total Time:10 minutes
Servings:4
Yield:4 servings

Nutrition Profile:

Suitable for Diabetes, Nut-Free, Dairy-Free, Low in Sodium, Soy-Free, High in Fiber, Heart-Healthy, Vegan, Vegetarian, Egg-Free, Gluten-Free, Low in Calories

Ingredients:

- 4 medium ears fresh corn, husked, or 10 oz. frozen whole-kernel corn, thawed
- 1 teaspoon olive oil
- 1 cup thin strips orange bell pepper
- 1 cup thinly sliced red onion
- ½ teaspoon kosher salt
- ¼ teaspoon ground pepper
- 2 tablespoons thinly sliced fresh basil for garnish

Directions:

1. Cut the kernels from the cobs to obtain 2 cups of corn.
2. Heat the olive oil in a 10-inch skillet over medium heat. Add the corn, bell pepper, and onion. Cook, stirring occasionally, until the bell pepper and onion reach a tender-crisp texture, approximately 5 minutes. Season with salt and pepper.
3. Serve the salad either warm or chilled. If chilling, drain excess liquid from the vegetables before refrigerating. Sprinkle with basil before serving, if desired.

Sheet-Pan Chicken Fajita Bowls

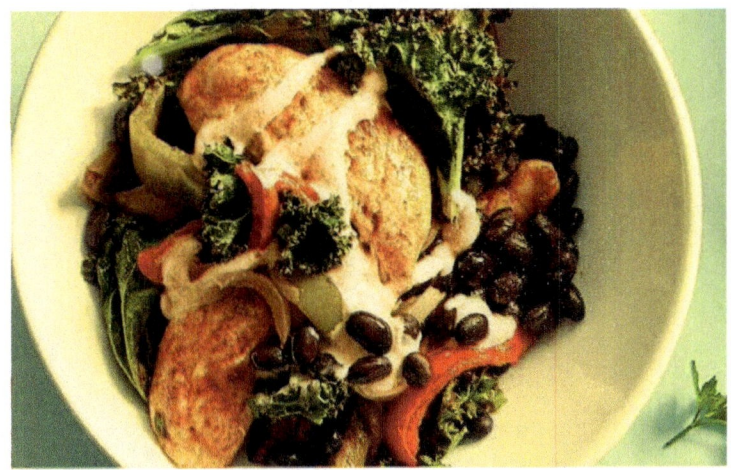

Preparation Time:20 minutes
Additional Time:20 minutes
Total Time:40 minutes
Servings:4
Yield:4 servings

Nutrition Profile:

Suitable for Diabetes, Nut-Free, Suitable for Healthy Pregnancy, Promotes Healthy Aging, Supports Healthy Immunity, Soy-Free, High in Fiber, High in Protein, Egg-Free, Gluten-Free, Low in Calories

Ingredients:

- 2 teaspoons chili powder
- 2 teaspoons ground cumin

- ¾ teaspoon salt, divided
- ½ teaspoon garlic powder
- ½ teaspoon smoked paprika
- ¼ teaspoon ground pepper
- 2 tablespoons olive oil, divided
- 1 ¼ pounds chicken tenders
- 1 medium yellow onion, sliced
- 1 medium red bell pepper, sliced
- 1 medium green bell pepper, sliced
- 4 cups chopped stemmed kale
- 1 (15 ounce) can no-salt-added black beans, rinsed
- ¼ cup low-fat plain Greek yogurt
- 1 tablespoon lime juice
- 2 teaspoons water

Directions:

1. Place a large rimmed baking sheet in the oven and preheat to 425 degrees F.
2. In a large bowl, combine chili powder, cumin, 1/2 teaspoon salt, garlic powder, paprika, and ground pepper. Transfer 1 teaspoon of the spice mixture to a medium bowl and set aside. Whisk 1 tablespoon of olive oil into the remaining spice mixture in the large bowl. Add chicken, onion, and red and green bell peppers; toss to coat.
3. Remove the pan from the oven and coat with cooking spray. Spread the chicken mixture evenly on the pan. Roast for 15 minutes.

4. Meanwhile, in a large bowl, combine kale and black beans with the remaining 1/4 teaspoon salt and 1 tablespoon olive oil; toss to coat.
5. Remove the pan from the oven. Stir the chicken and vegetables. Spread kale and beans evenly over the top. Roast until the chicken is cooked through and the vegetables are tender, for 5 to 7 minutes more.
6. Meanwhile, add yogurt, lime juice, and water to the reserved spice mixture; stir to combine.
7. Divide the chicken and vegetable mixture among 4 bowls. Drizzle with the yogurt dressing and serve.

Vegetable Weight-Loss Soup

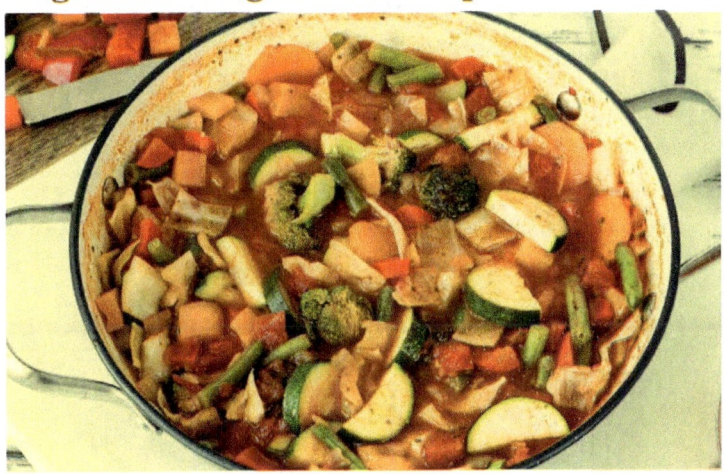

Active Time:45 minutes
Additional Time:15 minutes
Total Time:1 hour

Servings: 8
Yield: 8 servings

Nutrition Profile:
Suitable for Diabetes, Dairy-Free, Suitable for Healthy Aging, Supports Healthy Immunity, Low in Sodium, Soy-Free, Heart-Healthy, Egg-Free, Gluten-Free, Low-Calorie

Ingredients:

- 2 tablespoons extra-virgin olive oil
- 1 medium onion, chopped
- 2 medium carrots, chopped
- 2 stalks celery, chopped
- 12 ounces fresh green beans, cut into 1/2-inch pieces
- 2 cloves garlic, minced
- 8 cups no-salt-added chicken broth or low-sodium vegetable broth
- 2 (15 ounce) cans low-sodium cannellini or other white beans, rinsed
- 4 cups chopped kale
- 2 medium zucchini, chopped
- 4 Roma tomatoes, seeded and chopped
- 2 teaspoons red-wine vinegar
- ¾ teaspoon salt
- ½ teaspoon ground pepper
- 8 teaspoons prepared pesto

Directions:

1. Heat olive oil in a large pot over medium-high heat. Add onion, carrots, celery, green beans, and garlic. Cook, stirring frequently, until the vegetables begin to soften, approximately 10 minutes.
2. Add broth and bring to a boil. Reduce heat to a simmer and cook, stirring occasionally, until the vegetables are soft, about 10 minutes more.
3. Incorporate white beans, kale, zucchini, tomatoes, red-wine vinegar, salt, and pepper. Increase the heat to return to a simmer; cook until the zucchini and kale have softened, around 10 minutes.
4. Serve each portion of soup with 1 teaspoon of pesto on top.

Beef & Bean Sloppy Joes

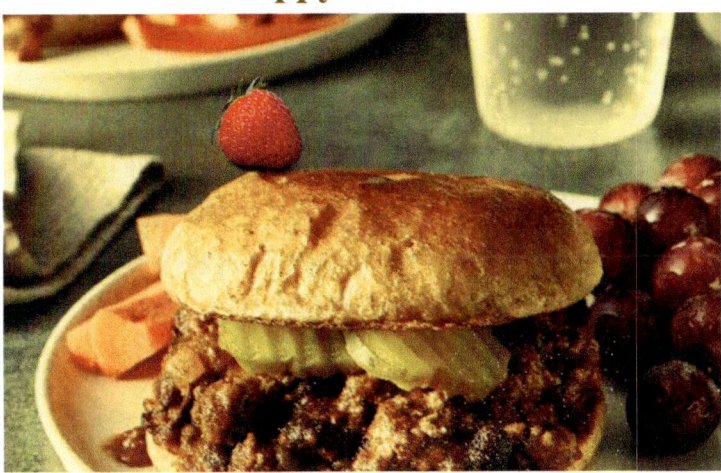

Preparation Time:20 minutes
Total Time:20 minutes

Servings: 4
Yield: 4 sandwiches

Nutrition Profile:
Suitable for Diabetes, Nut-Free, Dairy-Free, Suitable for Healthy Pregnancy, Promotes Healthy Aging, Supports Healthy Immunity, Low in Sodium, Suitable for High-Blood Pressure, High in Fiber, Heart-Healthy, Egg-Free, Low in Calories

Ingredients:

- 1 tablespoon extra-virgin olive oil
- 12 ounces 90%-lean ground beef
- 1 cup no-salt-added black beans, rinsed
- 1 cup chopped onion
- 2 teaspoons New Mexico chile powder
- ½ teaspoon garlic powder
- ½ teaspoon onion powder
- Pinch of cayenne pepper
- 1 cup no-salt-added tomato sauce
- 3 tablespoons ketchup
- 1 tablespoon reduced-sodium Worcestershire sauce
- 2 teaspoons spicy brown mustard
- 1 teaspoon light brown sugar
- 4 whole-wheat hamburger buns, split and toasted

Directions:

1. Heat olive oil in a large nonstick skillet over medium-high heat. Add beef and cook, breaking it up with a wooden spoon, until lightly browned but not completely cooked through, for 3 to 4 minutes. Using a slotted spoon, transfer the beef to a medium bowl, reserving drippings in the pan.
2. Add beans and onion to the pan; cook, stirring often, until the onion is softened, about 5 minutes. Add chile powder, garlic powder, onion powder, and cayenne; cook, stirring constantly, until fragrant, about 30 seconds. Stir in tomato sauce, ketchup, Worcestershire, mustard, and brown sugar. Return the beef to the pan. Bring to a simmer and cook, stirring often, until the beef is just cooked through and the sauce has thickened slightly, about 5 minutes. Serve on buns.

Chipotle-Lime Cauliflower Taco Bowls

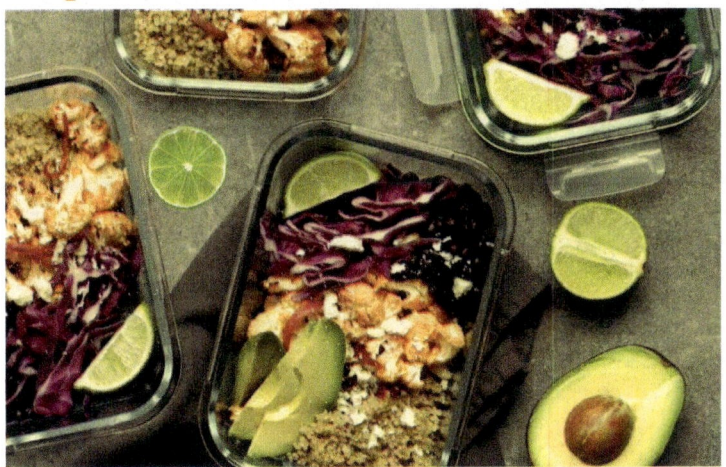

Preparation Time:20 minutes
Additional Time:20 minutes
Total Time:40 minutes
Servings:4
Yield:4 bowls

Nutrition Profile:

Suitable for Diabetes, Nut-Free, Suitable for Healthy Aging, Low in Sodium, Suitable for High-Blood Pressure, Soy-Free, High in Fiber, Heart-Healthy, Vegetarian, Egg-Free, Gluten-Free, Low in Calories

Ingredients:

- ¼ cup lime juice (from about 2 limes)
- 1-2 tablespoons chopped chipotles in adobo sauce
- 1 tablespoon honey
- 2 cloves garlic
- ½ teaspoon salt
- 1 small head cauliflower, cut into bite-size pieces
- 1 small red onion, halved and thinly sliced
- 2 cups cooked quinoa, cooled
- 1 cup no-salt-added canned black beans, rinsed
- ½ cup crumbled queso fresco
- 1 cup shredded red cabbage
- 1 medium avocado
- 1 lime, cut into 4 wedges (Optional)

Directions:

1. Preheat the oven to 450°F. Line a large rimmed baking sheet with foil.
2. In a blender, combine lime juice, chipotles to taste, honey, garlic, and salt. Process until mostly smooth. Place cauliflower in a large bowl; add the sauce and stir to coat. Transfer to the prepared baking sheet. Sprinkle onion over the cauliflower. Roast, stirring once, until the cauliflower is tender and browned in spots, 18 to 20 minutes; set aside to cool.
3. Divide quinoa among 4 single-serving lidded containers (1/2 cup each). Top each with one-fourth of the cauliflower mixture, 1/4 cup black beans, and 2 tablespoons cheese. Seal the containers and refrigerate for up to 4 days.
4. To reheat 1 container, vent the lid and microwave on High until steaming, 2 1/2 to 3 minutes. Top with 1/4 cup cabbage and 1/4 avocado (sliced). Serve with a lime wedge, if desired.

Vegetarian Stuffed Cabbage

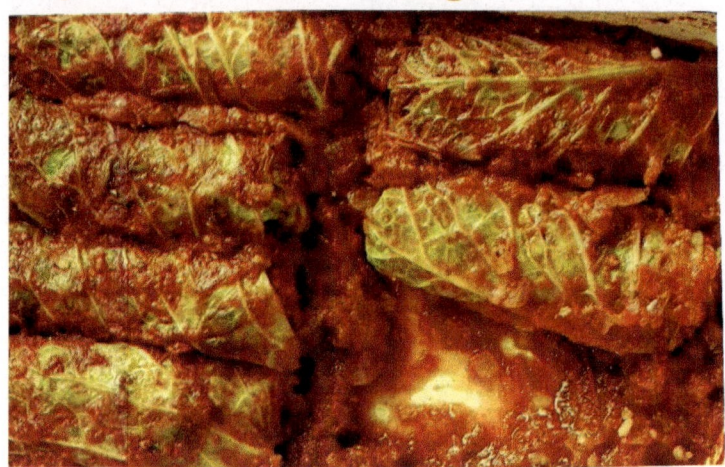

Cook Time:1 hour and 15 minutes
Additional Time:45 minutes
Total Time:2 hours
Servings:4
Yield:4 servings

Nutrition Profile:
Suitable for Diabetes, Dairy-Free, Suitable for Healthy Aging, Suitable for Healthy Immunity, Low in Sodium, Low in Added Sugar, Suitable for High-Blood Pressure, High in Fiber, Heart-Healthy, Vegan, Vegetarian, Gluten-Free, Low in Calories

Ingredients:

- 1 cup water
- ½ cup short-grain brown rice
- 1 teaspoon extra-virgin olive oil plus 2 tablespoons, divided
- 1 large Savoy cabbage (2-3 pounds)
- 1 pound baby bella mushrooms, finely chopped
- 1 large onion, finely chopped
- 4 cloves garlic, minced
- ½ teaspoon dried rubbed sage
- ½ teaspoon crumbled dried rosemary
- 1/2 teaspoon salt, divided
- 1/4 teaspoon freshly ground pepper plus 1/8 teaspoon, divided
- ½ cup red wine
- ¼ cup dried currants
- 1/3 cup toasted pine nuts, chopped
- 2 tablespoons extra-virgin olive oil, divided
- 1 small onion, chopped
- garlic, minced
- ¼ teaspoon salt
- ¼ teaspoon freshly ground pepper
- 1 28-ounce can no-salt-added crushed tomatoes
- ½ cup red wine

Directions:

1. Begin by cooking the rice: In a medium saucepan, combine water, rice, and 1 teaspoon of olive oil. Bring to a boil, then reduce heat to maintain a gentle simmer. Cover and cook until the water is absorbed and the rice is tender, about

40 to 50 minutes. Transfer the cooked rice to a large bowl and set aside.
2. While the rice cooks, prepare the cabbage and filling: Fill a large pot halfway with water and bring it to a boil. Line a baking sheet with a clean kitchen towel and place it nearby.
3. Core the Savoy cabbage and add it to the boiling water. Cook for 5 minutes, then use tongs to remove 8 large outer leaves as they soften. Place the leaves on the prepared baking sheet and pat them dry with more towels. Set aside.
4. Drain any remaining cabbage in a colander. Finely chop enough to yield about 3 cups and set aside.
5. In a large skillet, heat 1 1/2 tablespoons of olive oil over medium-high heat. Add mushrooms, onion, garlic, sage, rosemary, 1/4 teaspoon salt, and 1/4 teaspoon pepper. Cook until mushrooms release their juices and the pan becomes fairly dry, about 8 to 10 minutes. Stir in wine and cook until evaporated, about 3 minutes. Transfer the mixture to the bowl with cooked rice. Add currants and pine nuts.
6. In the same skillet, heat the remaining 1/2 tablespoon of oil over medium-high heat. Add chopped cabbage, 1/4 teaspoon salt, and 1/8 teaspoon pepper. Cook until cabbage wilts and begins to brown, about 3 to 5 minutes. Add to the rice mixture.
7. To prepare the sauce: In a separate large skillet, heat 1 tablespoon of oil over medium heat. Add onion, garlic, salt, and pepper. Cook until

softened, about 2 to 4 minutes. Add tomatoes and wine. Bring to a simmer and cook until slightly thickened, about 10 minutes.
8. Preheat the oven to 375 degrees F.
9. To assemble the stuffed cabbage: Place a cabbage leaf on a work surface and cut out the thick stem while keeping the leaf intact. Spoon about 3/4 cup of filling onto the center of each leaf. Fold both sides over the filling and roll up. Repeat with the remaining leaves and filling.
10. Spread 1 cup of the tomato sauce in a 9-by-13-inch baking dish. Arrange the stuffed cabbage rolls, seam side down, on top of the sauce. Pour the remaining sauce over the rolls and drizzle with the remaining 1 tablespoon of oil.
11. Bake, uncovered, basting twice with the sauce, until heated through, about 45 minutes.

Chicken Chili Verde

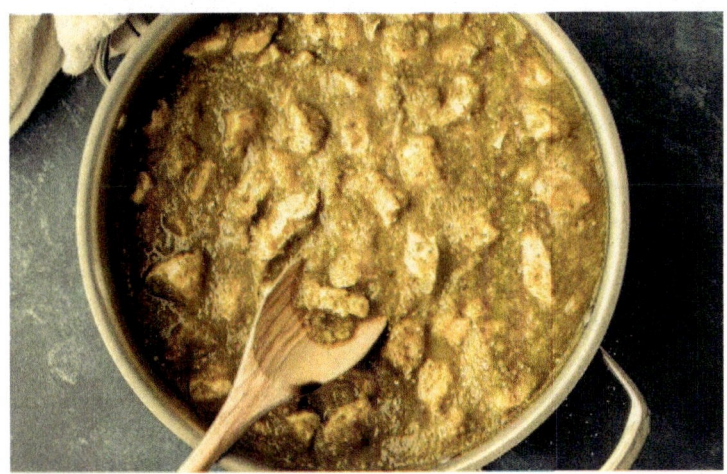

Active Time:30 minutes
Total Time:30 minutes
Servings:6
Yield:9 cups

Nutrition Profile:
Free from Nuts, Soy, High in Protein, Free from Eggs, Gluten-Free

Ingredients:

- 2 cans (15 ounces each) of pinto beans without added salt, rinsed and divided
- 1 tablespoon of canola oil
- 1 ½ pounds of boneless, skinless chicken thighs, trimmed and cut into bite-size pieces
- 2 cups of chopped yellow onion (equivalent to 1 medium onion)
- 2 cups of chopped poblano peppers (equivalent to 2 large peppers)
- 5 cloves of garlic, chopped (approximately 1 1/2 tablespoons)
- 4 cups of unsalted chicken stock
- 1 ½ cups of prepared salsa verde
- ½ teaspoon of salt
- 2 cups of frozen corn kernels (approximately 12 ounces)
- 2 cups of chopped spinach (approximately 2 ounces)
- 1 ½ cups of coarsely chopped fresh cilantro
- 6 tablespoons of sour cream

Directions:

1. In a small bowl, mash 1 cup of beans using a whisk or potato masher.
2. Heat the canola oil in a large heavy pot over high heat. Add the chicken and cook until browned, turning occasionally, for about 4 to 5 minutes.
3. Add the chopped onion, poblano peppers, and garlic to the pot. Cook until the onion becomes translucent and tender, which takes about 4 to 5 minutes.
4. Pour in the remaining whole beans, the mashed beans, chicken stock, salsa, and salt. Bring the mixture to a boil, then reduce the heat to medium and simmer until the chicken is fully cooked, approximately 3 minutes.
5. Stir in the frozen corn, chopped spinach, and cilantro. Continue to cook until the spinach wilts, which usually takes about 1 minute.
6. Serve the dish topped with sour cream.

Chickpea & Potato Curry

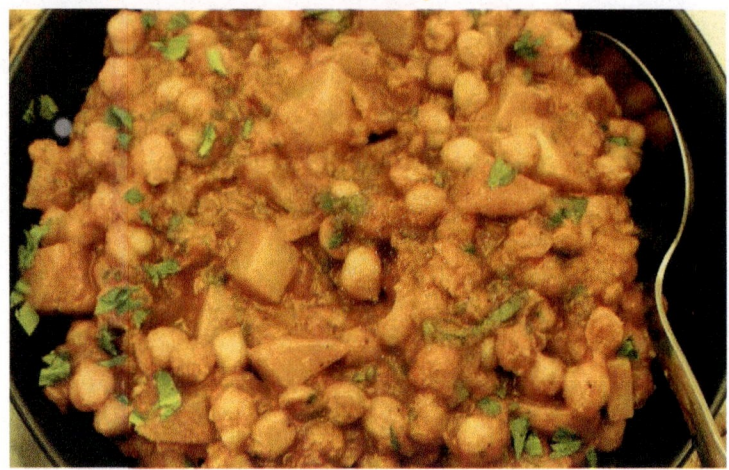

Preparation Time:35 minutes
Total Time:35 minutes
Servings:4
Yield:5 cups

Nutrition Profile:
Diabetes-Friendly, Low-Sodium, Low Added Sugar, Suitable for High-Blood Pressure, High in Fiber, Heart-Healthy, Vegan, Vegetarian, Low in Calories

Ingredients:

- 1 pound Yukon Gold potatoes, peeled and diced into 1-inch pieces
- 3 tablespoons grapeseed oil or canola oil
- 1 large onion, finely diced
- 3 cloves garlic, minced

- 2 teaspoons curry powder
- ¾ teaspoon salt
- ¼ teaspoon cayenne pepper
- 1 (14 ounce) can no-salt-added diced tomatoes
- ¾ cup water, divided
- 1 (15 ounce) can low-sodium chickpeas, rinsed
- 1 cup frozen peas
- ½ teaspoon garam masala

Directions:

1. Bring 1 inch of water to a boil in a large pot with a steamer basket. Add potatoes, cover, and steam until tender, approximately 6 to 8 minutes. Set aside the potatoes. Wipe the pot dry.
2. Heat oil in the pot over medium-high heat. Add onion and cook, stirring frequently, until soft and translucent, about 3 to 5 minutes. Incorporate garlic, curry powder, salt, and cayenne; cook, stirring constantly, for 1 minute. Add tomatoes and their juice; cook for an additional 2 minutes. Transfer the mixture to a blender or food processor. Add 1/2 cup water and blend until smooth.
3. Return the puree to the pot. Rinse the blender or food processor with the remaining 1/4 cup water and add to the pot along with the reserved potatoes, chickpeas, peas, and garam masala. Cook, stirring occasionally, until heated through, about 5 minutes.

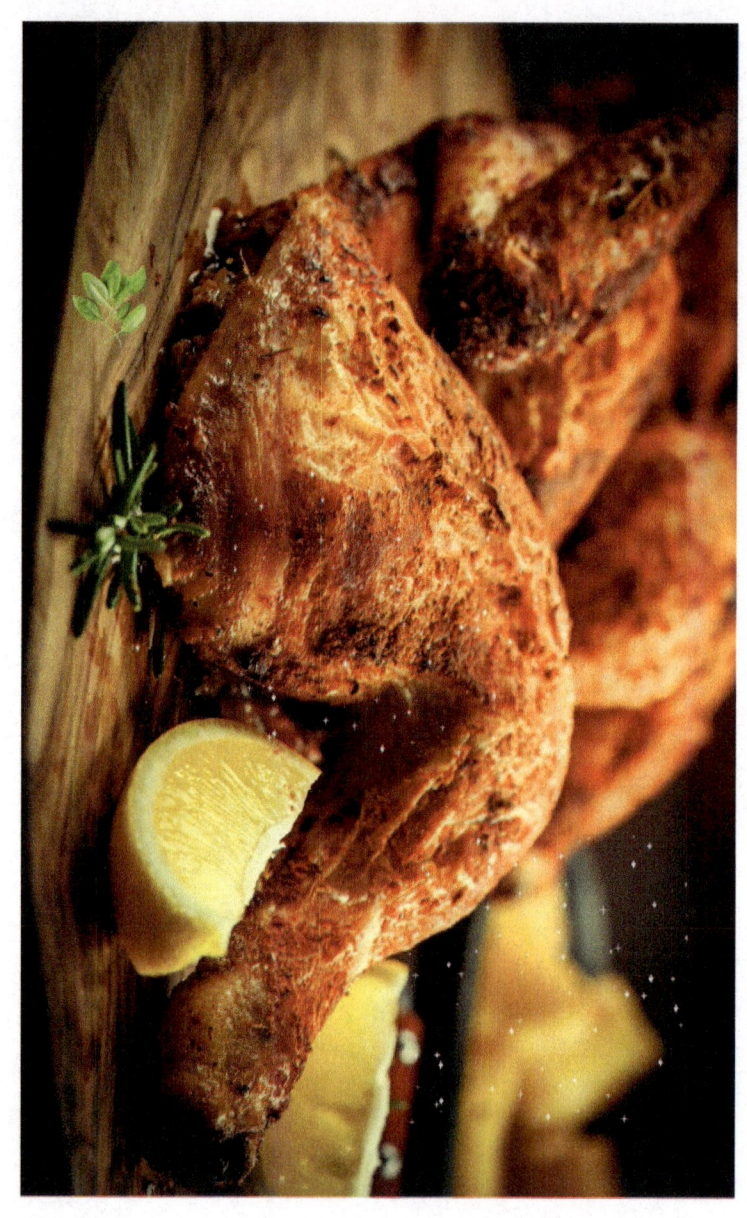

CHAPTER 3: DINNER RECIPES

Gochujang-Glazed Salmon with Garlic Spinach

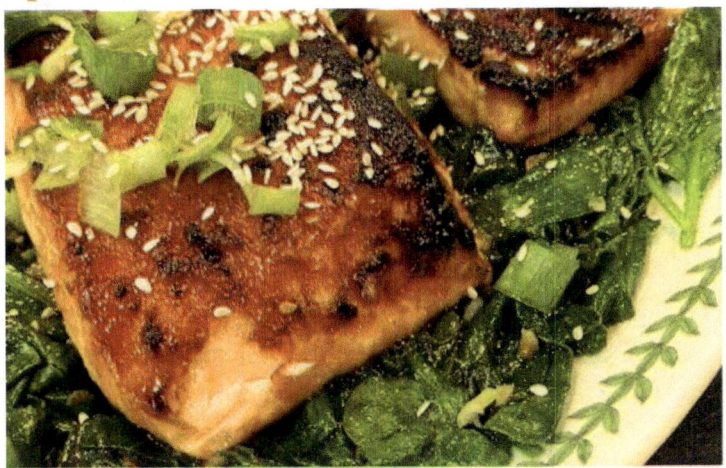

Preparation Time:20 minutes
Total Duration:20 minutes
Serves:4

Nutritional Profile:

Free from Nuts, Dairy, High in Protein, Heart-Friendly, Without Eggs, Low in Calories

Ingredients:

- 2 tablespoons of gochujang (Korean chili paste)
- 1 tablespoon of mirin (Japanese sweet rice wine)

- 2 tablespoons of low-sodium soy sauce, divided
- 1 tablespoon of honey
- 1 ½ teaspoons of toasted sesame oil, split
- 4 cloves of garlic, finely grated, separated
- 2 teaspoons of freshly grated ginger
- 1 ¼ pounds of salmon, ideally wild-caught, divided into four pieces
- 8 cups of baby spinach
- Sesame seeds and sliced green onions for topping

Instructions:

1. Set the oven rack to the upper third level and turn the broiler on high. Prepare a baking sheet with foil and lightly spray with cooking oil.
2. In a small mixing bowl, combine the gochujang, mirin, one tablespoon of the soy sauce, honey, half a teaspoon of sesame oil, a quarter of the grated garlic, and ginger to create a glaze. Dry the salmon pieces with a paper towel and arrange them skin-side down on the baking sheet. Apply the glaze evenly over the salmon. Broil the salmon until fully cooked, which should take between 5 to 8 minutes, depending on its thickness.
3. While the salmon is broiling, warm the remaining sesame oil in a large frying pan over medium-low heat. Add the rest of the garlic and sauté until it's aromatic and slightly golden, roughly 3 minutes. Introduce the spinach to the pan, stirring frequently until it has wilted and the excess moisture has evaporated, about 3 minutes. Take

the pan off the heat and mix in the remaining soy sauce.
4. To serve, place a generous amount of the garlicky spinach on a plate and top with a piece of broiled salmon. Garnish with sesame seeds and sliced green onions as desired

Chopped Salad with Chicken & Creamy Chipotle Dressing

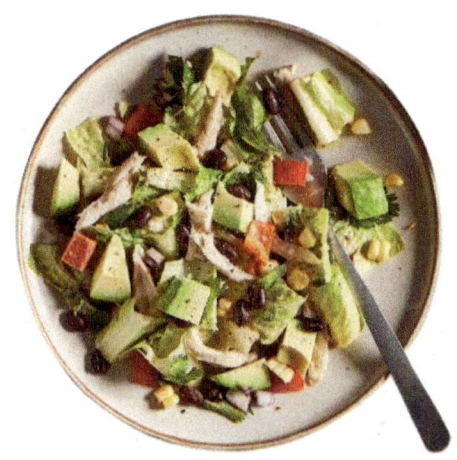

Preparation Time:15 minutes
Total Duration:15 minutes
Servings:6

Dietary Considerations:
Free from Nuts, Suitable for Healthy Pregnancy, Without Soy, High in Protein, Gluten-Free

Ingredients:

- 2 chipotle peppers in adobo sauce from a can
- ⅓ cup of mayonnaise
- ¼ cup of whole-milk Greek or skyr yogurt
- ¼ cup of fresh lime juice
- 1 garlic clove, minced
- ½ teaspoon of ground black pepper
- ½ teaspoon of cumin powder
- ¼ teaspoon of salt
- 1 can (15 ounces) of no-salt-added black beans, thoroughly rinsed
- 10 cups of chopped romaine lettuce
- 1 medium-sized red bell pepper, diced
- 2 small ears of corn, husks removed and kernels sliced off
- ½ cup of finely chopped red onion
- ½ cup of fresh cilantro, chopped
- 3 cups of shredded, cooked chicken breast
- 2 medium avocados, diced

Instructions:

1. In a blender, add the chipotle chiles, mayonnaise, yogurt, lime juice, minced garlic, ground pepper, cumin, and salt. Blend until the mixture is completely smooth, about 30 seconds.
2. In a large mixing bowl, combine the rinsed black beans, chopped romaine lettuce, diced red bell pepper, fresh corn kernels, chopped red onion, and chopped cilantro. Pour the previously

prepared dressing over this mixture and toss everything together until well-coated.
3. Serve the salad into 6 individual bowls. Top each bowl equally with the shredded chicken and diced avocado.

Lemongrass Pork & Spaghetti Squash Noodle Bowl with Peanut Sauce

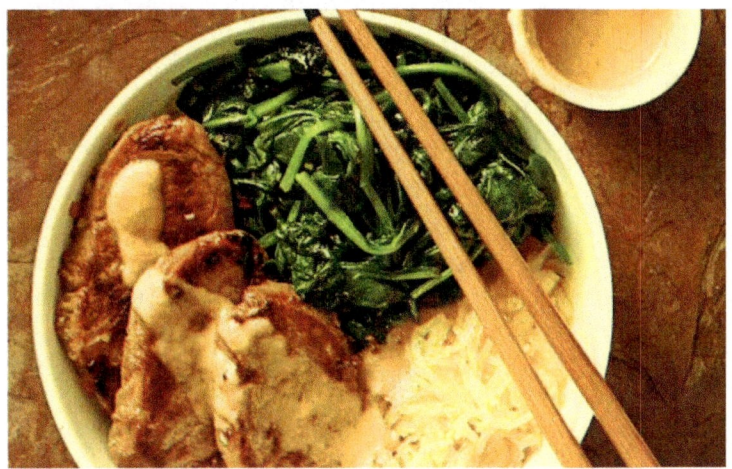

Cooking Time:45 minutes
Total Preparation Time:45 minutes
Servings:4
Yields:4 portions

Health Focus:

Dairy-Free, Suitable for Healthy Pregnancy, Promotes Healthy Aging and Immunity, High in Protein, Gluten-Free, Low in Calories

Ingredients:

- 2 tablespoons of finely chopped fresh ginger, split use
- 2 tablespoons of finely chopped fresh lemongrass
- 2 tablespoons of light brown sugar
- 2 tablespoons of low-sodium soy sauce
- 1 tablespoon of fish sauce
- 1 pound of pork tenderloin, sliced into 1/2-inch pieces
- 1 spaghetti squash, ranging from 2 1/2 to 3 pounds, halved and deseeded
- 3 tablespoons of peanut oil, used separately
- 1 pound of fresh baby spinach
- ½ cup of light coconut milk
- ¼ cup of smooth natural peanut butter
- ¼ cup of water

Instructions:

1. In a shallow bowl, mix together 1 tablespoon of ginger, lemongrass, brown sugar, soy sauce, and fish sauce. Add the pork slices, ensuring they're well coated with the mixture. Allow to marinate for 20 minutes, turning occasionally.
2. For the spaghetti squash, place it cut-side down in a microwave-safe dish and add 2 tablespoons of water. Microwave on high until tender, about 10 minutes. Alternatively, you can bake the squash halves cut-side down in a preheated oven at 400 degrees F until soft, which takes about 40 to 50 minutes.

3. In a large skillet, heat 2 tablespoons of peanut oil over medium-high heat. Stir in the remaining ginger and gradually add the spinach, cooking until wilted, which should take about 1 to 2 minutes. Move the spinach to a plate and cover to keep warm.
4. Clean the skillet, then heat the last tablespoon of peanut oil over medium-high heat. Add the marinated pork (including the marinade) and sear, turning once, until browned on both sides, roughly 2 minutes per side. Move the pork to the plate with the spinach, keeping it covered, and leaving the pan juices.
5. To the skillet, add coconut milk, peanut butter, and ¼ cup water. Stir well, loosening any browned bits from the pan, and cook for about a minute.
6. To serve, fork-shred the spaghetti squash into bowls. Drizzle each serving with 2 tablespoons of the peanut sauce, then add the pork and spinach. Finish by drizzling the remaining sauce over the top.

Kale & Avocado Salad with Blueberries & Edamame

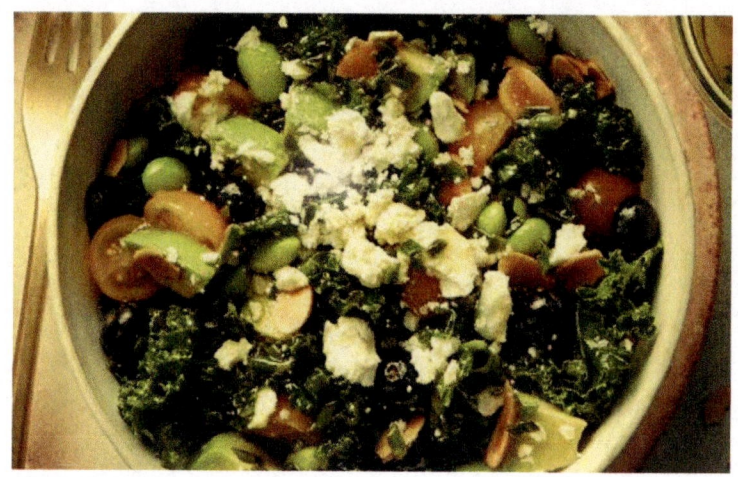

Preparation Time:20 minutes
Total Duration:20 minutes
Number of Servings:4
Total Yield:8 cups

Suitable For:
Diabetes-Friendly, Supports Healthy Pregnancy,

Vegetarian, Free from Eggs and Gluten

Ingredients:

- 6 cups of curly kale, stems removed and roughly chopped
- 1 diced avocado
- 1 cup of blueberries
- 1 cup of yellow cherry tomatoes, cut in halves

- 1 cup of cooked and shelled edamame
- ¼ cup of sliced almonds, toasted
- ½ cup of goat cheese, crumbled (equivalent to 2 ounces)
- ¼ cup of olive oil
- 3 tablespoons of fresh lemon juice
- 1 tablespoon of finely chopped chives
- 1 ½ teaspoons of honey
- 1 teaspoon of Dijon mustard
- 1 teaspoon of salt

Instructions:

1. In a large mixing bowl, add the kale. Use your hands to gently massage the leaves until they begin to soften. Incorporate the diced avocado, blueberries, cherry tomatoes, edamame, almonds, and crumbled goat cheese into the kale.
2. For the dressing, mix the olive oil, lemon juice, chives, honey, mustard, and salt in a small bowl or a jar with a secure lid. Whisk together or shake until thoroughly combined.
3. Pour the prepared vinaigrette over the salad ingredients. Toss everything together to ensure the salad is evenly coated with the dressing.

Teriyaki Chicken Skillet Casserole with Broccoli

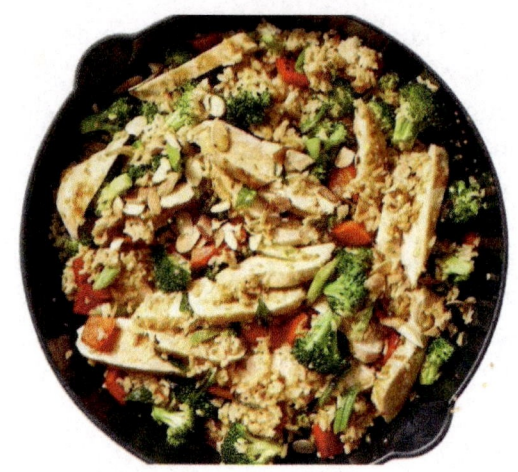

Preparation Time: 15 minutes
Total Cooking Time: 30 minutes
Number of Servings: 6

Suitable for:

Diabetes-Friendly, Dairy-Free, Heart-Healthy, High-Protein, Egg-Free

Ingredients:

- 2 tablespoons of sesame oil
- 3 cups of small broccoli florets (about 7 ounces)
- 1 cup of chopped red bell pepper
- 1 cup of chopped green onions (roughly 5 scallions)
- 1/3 cup of low-sodium teriyaki sauce
- 1/4 cup of water

- 2 tablespoons of cornstarch
- 2 minced garlic cloves
- 3 cups of sliced precooked chicken
- 3 cups of cooked brown rice
- Optional garnish: Toasted sesame seeds or toasted almond slices

Instructions:

1. Start by heating your oven to 350°F (175°C).
2. In a large skillet that's safe for oven use, warm the sesame oil over medium heat. Toss in the broccoli, red bell pepper, and green onions. Stir and cook until they begin to soften, about 3 to 5 minutes.
3. In a mixing cup, whisk together the teriyaki sauce, water, cornstarch, and minced garlic. Pour this mixture into the skillet, adding the sliced chicken and brown rice as well. Stir everything together until fully mixed.
4. Move the skillet to the preheated oven. Bake for approximately 15 minutes, or until the dish is heated through and the vegetables have reached your desired tenderness.
5. Upon serving, consider garnishing with toasted sesame seeds or almond slices for an added touch, if you like.

Spicy Shrimp Tacos

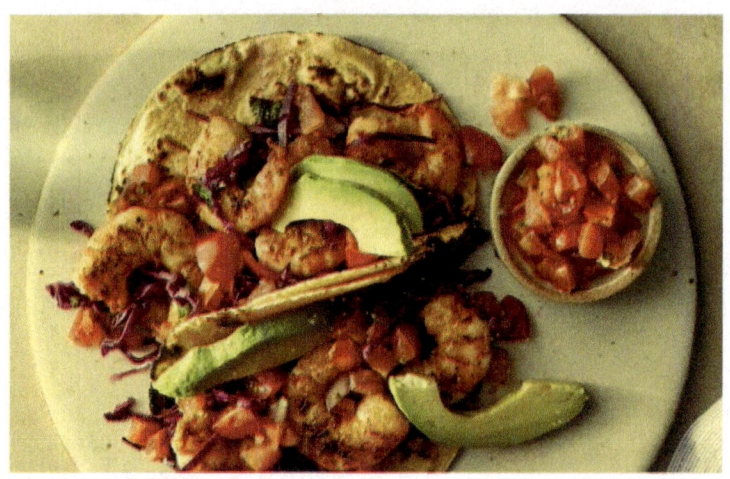

Preparation Time:20 minutes
Total Cooking Duration:20 minutes
Servings:4
Total Yield:8 tacos

Dietary Considerations:

Free from nuts, dairy, soy, eggs, and gluten; High in protein, suitable for healthy aging and boosting immunity.

Ingredients:

- 4 tablespoons of high-quality extra-virgin olive oil, split
- 1 pound of large shrimp, cleaned and deveined
- 1 tablespoon of Shrimp Seasoning
- A pinch (⅛ teaspoon) of salt
- 1 ½ cups of red cabbage, cut into thin strips

- 2 tablespoons of freshly chopped cilantro
- 2 tablespoons of fresh lime juice
- 8 corn tortillas (6-inch), warmed
- 1 ripe avocado, cut into slices
- ½ cup of fresh pico de gallo

Instructions:

1. In a large frying pan, heat up 2 tablespoons of olive oil over a high setting. Season the shrimp with the shrimp seasoning and a pinch of salt, ensuring an even coating. Place the seasoned shrimp in the skillet and cook, frequently stirring, until they turn opaque and are thoroughly cooked, about 3 to 4 minutes. Once done, move the shrimp to a separate dish.
2. In a medium-sized bowl, combine the sliced red cabbage, chopped cilantro, lime juice, and the remaining 2 tablespoons of olive oil. Stir the mixture until everything is well-coated.
3. Assemble the tacos by distributing the cooked shrimp evenly amongst the warmed corn tortillas. Follow by adding a generous helping of the cabbage mixture on top of the shrimp. Finish each taco with a few slices of avocado and a spoonful of pico de gallo.

Roasted Brussels Sprout & Butternut Squash Salad

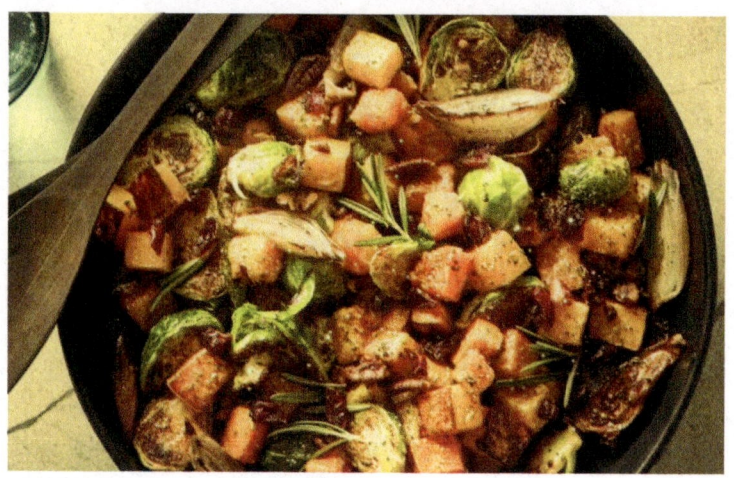

Preparation Time:15 minutes
Additional Time:40 minutes
Total Duration:55 minutes
Portions:4
Output: 5 cups

Health Profile:

Excludes nuts, dairy, soy, eggs, and gluten; High in fiber, suitable for vegans and vegetarians, supports immune health.

Ingredients:

- 4 ½ cups of butternut squash, chopped into 3/4-inch pieces

- 3 medium shallots, each cut into quarters
- 4 ½ teaspoons of olive oil, split
- 1 pound of Brussels sprouts, halved or quartered if extra large
- ½ teaspoon of salt, split
- 1 tablespoon plus 1 1/2 teaspoons of sherry vinegar
- 1 tablespoon of tahini
- 1 teaspoon of genuine maple syrup
- 1 teaspoon of freshly minced rosemary
- ½ teaspoon of ground black pepper
- ⅓ cup of dried cranberries
- ⅓ cup of toasted and chopped pecans or walnuts (optional)

Instructions:

1. Start by heating your oven to 425 degrees F. On a broad, edged baking tray, mix the squash pieces and quartered shallots with 1 1/2 teaspoons of olive oil, ensuring they are evenly coated. Place in the oven to roast until they are nearly tender and begin to brown, about 20 minutes.
2. In the meantime, mix the Brussels sprouts with 1 1/2 teaspoons of olive oil and a pinch of 1/4 teaspoon salt in a separate bowl, making sure they are evenly coated.
3. Once the initial roasting period is done, remove the baking tray from the oven. Combine the Brussels sprouts with the squash and shallots, spreading them out to form an even layer. Put

back in the oven to roast until every vegetable is tender and has a golden-brown color, roughly 20 minutes more.
4. While waiting, in a small mixing bowl, combine the sherry vinegar, tahini, maple syrup, chopped rosemary, black pepper, and the rest of the olive oil and salt. Whisk together well.
5. After roasting, transfer the vegetables into a large mixing bowl. Mix in the dried cranberries and the previously prepared dressing, tossing until everything is nicely coated. Optionally, you can add chopped nuts for an extra crunch.
6. This dish can be served straight away or left to stand at room temperature for up to 4 hours for flavors to meld. For storing, keep in a sealed container in the fridge for up to two days, and allow it to reach room temperature for 30 minutes before serving again.

Slow-Cooker Chicken Chili

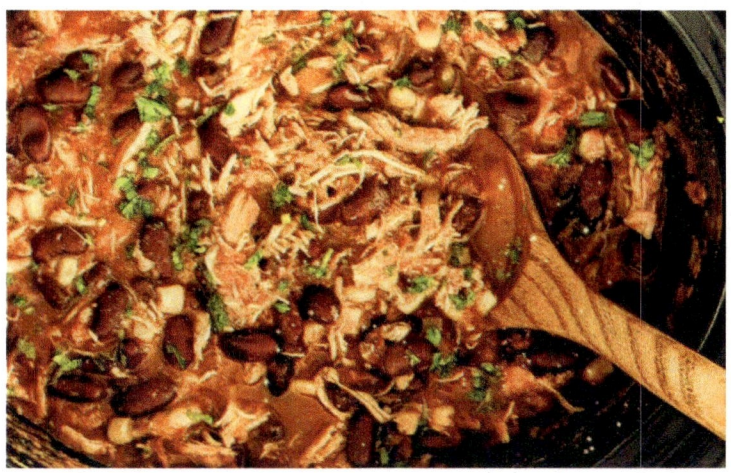

Preparation Time:25 minutes
Total Cooking Time:3 hours and 25 minutes
Serves:8

Health Considerations:

Suitable for diabetics, free from nuts, soy, eggs, and gluten; beneficial for heart health and high in protein.

Ingredients:

- 2 cups of unsalted chicken stock
- 1 can (28 ounces) of no-salt-added crushed tomatoes
- 2 cans (15 ounces each) of no-salt-added dark kidney beans, washed and drained
- 1 medium yellow onion, diced
- 1 medium red bell pepper, diced
- 6 cloves of garlic, minced

- 1 tablespoon of finely minced chipotle chili in adobo sauce, plus 1 tablespoon of the sauce
- 2 teaspoons of ground cumin
- 1 teaspoon of ground coriander
- 1 teaspoon of dried oregano
- 1 teaspoon of salt
- 1.5 pounds of boneless, skinless chicken breasts
- 3 tablespoons of fresh lime juice
- ¾ cup of shredded sharp Cheddar cheese
- 2 medium avocados, diced
- ⅓ cup of fresh cilantro, chopped

Instructions:

1. In a 5-quart slow cooker, combine the chicken stock, crushed tomatoes, kidney beans, chopped onion, diced bell pepper, minced garlic, chipotle chili, adobo sauce, cumin, coriander, oregano, and salt. Mix well.
2. Place the chicken breasts into the mixture in the slow cooker, ensuring they are completely submerged. Cover with the lid and cook until a thermometer inserted into the thickest part of the chicken reads 165°F. This should take approximately 3 hours on the High setting or 4 to 5 hours on Low.
3. Carefully remove the chicken to a chopping board and allow it to cool for about 5 minutes. Then, shred the chicken using two forks and return the shredded meat to the slow cooker. Stir in the lime juice thoroughly.

4. Serve the chili in 8 individual bowls, garnishing each with shredded Cheddar cheese, diced avocado, and chopped cilantro before serving.

Chicken Enchilada Skillet Casserole

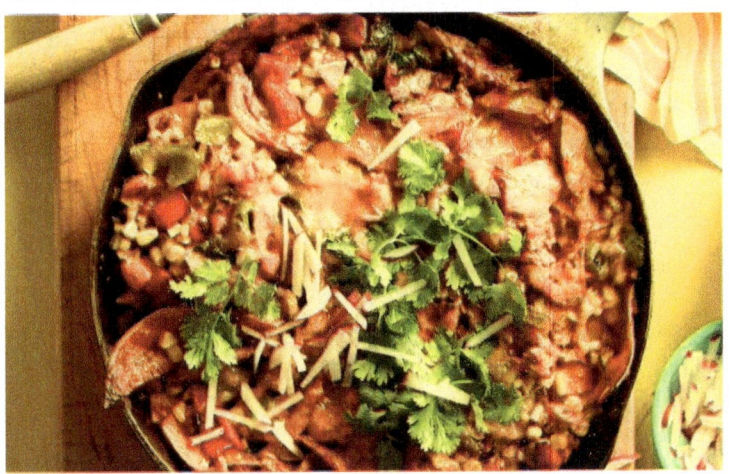

Active Preparation Time: 25 minutes
Overall Cooking Time: 40 minutes
Servings: 6

Health Benefits:
Suitable for those managing diabetes, high in protein

Ingredients:

- 2 tablespoons of olive oil
- 1 cup of either fresh or frozen corn kernels

- ½ cup of diced green bell pepper
- ½ cup of diced red bell pepper
- ½ cup of diced onion
- One 5-ounce packet of baby spinach
- 2 ½ cups of shredded, previously cooked chicken breast
- One 8-ounce package of either red or green enchilada sauce (brand example: Frontera)
- 1 ¼ cups of store-bought, fresh salsa
- Eight corn tortillas (5- or 6-inch), sliced into 1-inch strips
- 1 ½ cups of shredded, low-fat Cheddar cheese
- 1 cup of roughly chopped grape tomatoes
- ¼ cup of freshly chopped cilantro
- ¼ cup of radishes cut into matchsticks

Instructions:

1. Begin by heating your oven to 350°F (175°C).
2. In a large, oven-safe skillet, such as one made of cast iron, heat the olive oil. Add the corn, green and red bell peppers, and onion to the skillet. Cook these, stirring them now and then, until they start to char, which should take about 7 to 10 minutes. Slowly incorporate the baby spinach, adding it in portions; stir frequently until the spinach has wilted, roughly 1 to 2 minutes.
3. Mix in the shredded chicken, enchilada sauce, and salsa until everything is well combined. Carefully fold in the strips of tortilla, then evenly sprinkle the cheese on top. Move the skillet to the

oven and bake until the cheese is bubbly and golden, which will take around 15 minutes.
4. Once baked, garnish the casserole with the grape tomatoes, chopped cilantro, and matchstick-cut radishes before serving.

Sheet-Pan Balsamic-Parmesan Roasted Chickpeas & Vegetables

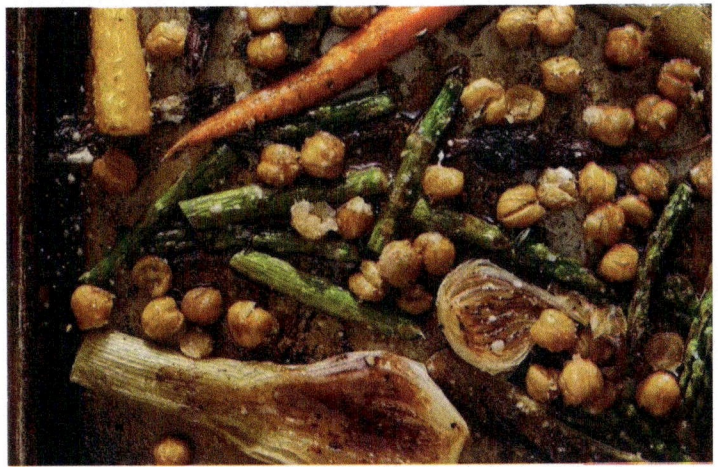

Preparation Time:15 minutes
Additional Cooking Time:25 minutes
Total Recipe Time:40 minutes
Number of Servings:4
Volume Yielded:4 cups

Health Benefits:

Supports bone health, suitable for diabetes management, free from nuts, promotes healthy aging and immunity, low in sodium and added sugars, soy-free, rich in fiber, good for heart health, vegetarian, without eggs or gluten.

Ingredients:

- One 15-ounce can of chickpeas without added salt, thoroughly rinsed
- 8 ounces of multicolored mini carrots, tops trimmed and peeled
- 2 bunches of spring onions, greens removed, bulbs sliced in half lengthwise
- 6 tablespoons of extra-virgin olive oil, used separately
- ¼ teaspoon of salt, divided into portions
- 8 ounces of asparagus, chopped into 2-inch segments
- ½ cup of finely grated Parmesan cheese
- 2 tablespoons of balsamic vinegar
- 1 teaspoon of honey
- ½ teaspoon of Dijon mustard
- ½ teaspoon of freshly ground black pepper
- 1 teaspoon of fresh thyme leaves

Instructions:

1. Position a large rimmed baking sheet in the center of the oven and preheat it to 400 degrees F. Use another baking sheet lined with paper towels. Spread the chickpeas on this lined sheet, patting them dry and rubbing gently with additional paper towels to peel off the skins. Dispose of the skins.

2. Move the skinless chickpeas to a sizable bowl. Mix in the baby carrots, spring onions, half of the olive oil (3 tablespoons), and half of the salt (1/8 teaspoon), ensuring an even coating. Lay this mixture flat on the preheated baking sheet. Roast until the veggies achieve a golden-brown color and softness, roughly 30 minutes, stirring once midway. Introduce asparagus in the final 10 minutes of roasting. Afterward, evenly distribute Parmesan over the veggies and roast for another 5 minutes until the cheese has melted.
3. While the vegetables roast, prepare the dressing by combining the balsamic vinegar, honey, mustard, black pepper, and the remaining olive oil and salt in a small bowl. After roasting, drizzle this balsamic dressing over the vegetables and garnish with fresh thyme leaves. Serve hot

28 DAYS MEAL PLAN

This plan focuses on high-protein, heart-healthy, diabetes-appropriate, high-fiber, vegetarian, and gluten-free options.

Week 1

Day 1

- Breakfast: Avocado Toast on Gluten-Free Bread
- Lunch: Roasted Vegetable Salad with Balsamic Dressing
- Dinner: Slow Cooker Chicken Chili

Day 2

- Breakfast: Oatmeal with Fresh Berries and Honey
- Lunch: Quinoa Salad with Chickpeas and Spring Vegetables
- Dinner: Shrimp Tacos with Cabbage Slaw

Day 3

- Breakfast: Smoothie with Spinach, Banana, and Protein Powder
- Lunch: Butternut Squash and Brussels Sprouts with Tahini Dressing
- Dinner: Chicken and Vegetable Enchilada Casserole

Day 4

- Breakfast: Scrambled Eggs with Spinach and Feta (use plant-based eggs for vegan)
- Lunch: Mediterranean Chickpea Salad
- Dinner: Grilled Fish with Quinoa and Steamed Broccoli

Day 5

- Breakfast: Yogurt with Granola and Mixed Fruit
- Lunch: Lentil Soup with Spinach and Tomatoes
- Dinner: Vegetable Stir-Fry with Tofu over Brown Rice

Day 6

- Breakfast: Pancakes made with Almond Flour, topped with Maple Syrup
- Lunch: Avocado and Black Bean Wrap (use gluten-free wrap)
- Dinner: Baked Salmon with Roasted Asparagus and Wild Rice

Day 7

- Breakfast: Chia Pudding with Coconut Milk and Mixed Berries
- Lunch: Kale Salad with Roasted Chickpeas, Avocado, and Lemon Dressing
- Dinner: Vegetarian Chili

Week 2

Repeat Week 1 for simplicity and to minimize food waste, adjusting as desired for variety or to incorporate seasonal ingredients.

Week 3 & 4

For Weeks 3 and 4, consider revisiting the meals from Weeks 1 and 2, perhaps introducing one or two new recipes to each week for variety. Experiment with different seasonings and dressings to modify dishes slightly and keep the meal plan exciting. For example, try adding new protein sources to salads or substituting different vegetables in the stir-fry and casseroles based on availability and preference.

Additional Tips:

- Snacks: Include healthy snacks such as nuts, fruits, and vegetables with hummus between meals to maintain energy levels.
- Hydration: Drink plenty of water throughout the day to stay hydrated.
- Customization: Adjust portion sizes according to individual dietary needs and activity levels.
- Meal Prep: Consider preparing some meals in advance to save time during busy days.

CONVERSION TABLE

Volume Conversions:

1 teaspoon (tsp) = 5 milliliters (ml)
1 tablespoon (tbsp) = 15 milliliters (ml)
1 fluid ounce (oz) = 30 milliliters (ml)

1 cup (c) = 240 milliliters (ml)
1 pint (pt) = 473 milliliters (ml)
1 quart (qt) = 946 milliliters (ml)
1 gallon (gal) = 3.785 liters (l)

Weight Conversions:
1 ounce (oz) = 28.35 grams (g)
1 pound (lb) = 453.59 grams (g)
1 kilogram (kg) = 2.205 pounds (lb)

Temperature Conversions:
Fahrenheit to Celsius: (°F - 32) × 5/9 = °C
Celsius to Fahrenheit: (°C × 9/5) + 32 = °F

Common Equivalents:
1 stick of butter = 1/2 cup = 8 tablespoons = 113 grams
1 cup of flour = 120 grams
1 cup of sugar = 200 grams
Feel free to customize and expand this table based on your specific needs.

Time Conversions:
1 minute (min) = 60 seconds (s)
1 hour (hr) = 60 minutes (min)

Length Conversions:
1 inch (in) = 2.54 centimeters (cm)
1 foot (ft) = 30.48 centimeters (cm)
1 yard (yd) = 0.914 meters (m)
1 meter (m) = 39.37 inches (in)

Common Oven Temperatures:
Slow or Low Heat: 300°F (150°C)
Moderate Heat: 350°F (180°C)
Moderate to Hot Heat: 375°F (190°C)
Hot: 400°F (200°C)
Very Hot: 450°F (230°C)

Liquid Measurements:
1 standard cup = 8 fluid ounces = 240 milliliters
1 standard tablespoon = 1/2 fluid ounce = 15 milliliters
1 standard teaspoon = 1/6 fluid ounce = 5 milliliters

Metric to Imperial Conversions:
1 centimeter (cm) = 0.3937 inches (in)
1 meter (m) = 1.0936 yards (yd)
1 liter (l) = 1.76 pints
1 milliliter (ml) = 0.034 fluid ounces

Printed in Great Britain
by Amazon

39836728R00046